KETO Comfort Food

Amanda Miller

1

Table of Contents

Introduction 6

Chapter 1. Breakfast Recipes 13

1   Lemon Crepes 14

2   Turkey Bacon & Spinach Crepes...................... 15

3   Bacon Quiche with Cheddar Cheese 17

4   Perfect Buttermilk Pancakes............................ 18

5   Ginger Pancakes 20

Chapter 2. Snack & Appetizer Recipes...................... 23

6   Chicken and Spinach Meatballs....................... 24

7   Deviled Eggs 25

8   Cauliflower Bites... 26

9   Romano and Asiago Cheese Crisps................ 27

10   Caprese Sticks 28

Chapter 3. Poultry Recipes 29

11   Ginger Turkey Drumsticks Curry................... 30

12   Roasted Chicken Breasts with Capers 31

13   Stuffed Chicken Breasts with Cucumber
Noodle Salad.. 33

14   Creamy Stuffed Chicken with Parma Ham ..35

15   Chicken Wings with Herb Chutney 36

Chapter 4. Beef.. 39

16   Balsamic Skirt Steak.................................40

17   Beef & Cheddar Stuffed Eggplants..............42

18   Sweet Chipotle Grilled Beef Ribs 43

19   Lemony Beef Rib Roast 44

20   Grilled Sirloin Steak with Sauce Diane.........46

Chapter 5. Pork Recipes 49

21   Chili Pork Stew...50

22   Pork Fillet and Tomato Salad.......................51

23   Peanut Butter Pork Stir-Fry 52

24   Hot Pork with Dill Pickles 53

25   Pork Casserole...54

Chapter 6. Fish and Seafood 57

26   Cheese Shrimp 58

27   Rosemary Scallops.....................................59

28   Swai Fish Fillets in Port Wine......................60

29   Red Cabbage Tilapia Bowl 62

30   Sicilian-Style Sardines with Zoodles.............63

Chapter 8. Vegetable Recipes.......................65

31   Chinese Cauliflower Rice with Eggs 66

32   Mushroom Stroganoff 67

33   Zucchini Fritters 68

34   Cheese Stuffed Spaghetti Squash................69

35   Herbed Eggplant and Kale Bake 71

Chapter 7. Salad Recipes 73

36   Shrimp & Avocado Cauliflower Salad 74

37   Broccoli Slaw Salad with Mustard Vinaigrette 75

38   Pork Burger Salad with Yellow Cheddar 76

39   Warm Baby Artichoke Salad 77

40   Spinach & Turnip Salad with Bacon 78

Chapter 8. Soup Recipes 81

41   Herby Cheese & Bacon Soup 82

42   Spring Vegetable Soup 84

43   Wild Mushroom Soup 85

44   Creamy Chicken Soup 86

45   Creamy Feta Soup 87

Chapter 9. Dessert Recipes 89

46   Strawberries Coated with Chocolate Chips. 90

47   Cream Cheese Chocolate Cake 91

48   Mocha Mousse 93

49   Flaxseed Coconut Bread Pudding 95

50   Strawberry Mousse 99

Introduction

A keto diet is an eating plan focused on foods that offer a high amount of healthful fat, moderate level of protein, and very low carbohydrates. People who say they are on a 'keto diet' are people who ensure that their regular food intake contains a lot of healthful fat, an adequate amount of protein, and very low carbohydrates. This means their dietary macronutrients are divided into about 55% to 60% fat, 30% to 35% protein, and 5% to 10% carbohydrate. In the end, the goal of the keto diet is to get more energy from healthful fats than from carbohydrates.

How Does It Work?

Your body makes use of any energy source it finds readily available, which is often glucose converted from carbohydrates. By increasing the level of healthful fat you take and reducing your carbohydrate intake, your glycogen level depletes, which forces your body to go through metabolic changes. Two metabolic processes occur when your body stores low-level carbohydrates. They are called gluconeogenesis and ketogenesis.

Glycogenesis is the production of glucose in your body, and when the glucose production level stops due to low carbohydrate level, the production of glucose becomes too low to keep up with the needs of your body, which forces your body to adapt to ketogenesis as an alternative. Ketogenesis begins to produce energy for your body, and ketone bodies become your body's primary source of energy, which is known as the 'ketosis state' that continues to be as long as your body is deprived of carbohydrates. Because your body is deprived of carbohydrates, which is primarily the cause of weight gain, your body can burn fat faster and convert the available fat into energy.

The ketone bodies are integrated into your body system and are used to produce energy through the heart, muscle tissue, and kidneys and also cross the blood-brain barrier to be an alternative source of energy to the brain.

The Ketosis

Switching to a high-fat moderate protein cycle, your liver has now a new "fuel boss" - the fat. Once your liver begins preparing your body for the fuel change, the fat from the liver will start producing ketones – hence the name Ketogenic. What glucose is for the carbs, the ketones are for the fat, meaning they are the tiny molecules created once the fat is broken down to be used as energy. The switch from glucose to ketones is something that has pushed many people away from this diet. Some people consider this to be a dangerous process, but the truth is, your body will run just as efficiently on ketones as it does on glucose.

Once your body shifts to using ketones as fuel, you are in the state of ketosis. Ketosis is a metabolic process that may be interpreted as a little 'shock' to your body. However, this is far from dangerous. Every change in life requires adaptation, and so does this. This adaptation process is not set in stone, and every person goes through ketosis differently. However, for most people, it takes around 2 weeks to fully adapt to the new lifestyle.

Note! This is all biological and completely healthy. You have spent your whole life packing your body with glucose; naturally, you need time to adapt to the new dietary change.

Keto Flu

The term Keto flu describes a very common experience for new ketoers, but it often goes away in the first week. When starting with keto, you may have some slight discomfort or feel fatigued, headache, nausea, cramps, etc.

The reasons Keto flu occurs are two:

1.Keto diet is diuretic; therefore you visit the bathroom quite often, which leads to the loss of electrolytes and water. The solution is either drinking more water or a bouillon cube, to replenish electrolytes reserves. I suggest that you also increase the consumption of potassium, magnesium. calcium, and phosphorus.

2.Shifting to Keto is at first a big shock for the body. The reason is that it's designed to process carbs and now there are almost none. You may feel increased fatigue, nausea, etc. The solution is to decrease carbs intake gradually.

What To Eat

Certain foods will help you up to your fat intake and provide you with more longer-lasting energy: Meats, Eggs, Fish and Seafood, Bacon, Sausage, Cacao, and sugar-free chocolate, Avocado, and berries, Leafy Greens - all of them, Vegetables: cucumber, zucchini, asparagus, broccoli, onion, Brussel sprout, cabbage, tomato, eggplants, seaweed, peppers, squash, Full-Fat Dairy (heavy cream, yogurt, sour cream, cheese, etc.); Nuts — nuts are packed with healthy fats, chestnuts, and cashews, as they contain more carbs than the rest of the nuts. Macadamia nuts, walnuts pecans, and almonds are the best for the Keto diet.; Seeds - chia, flaxseeds, sunflower seeds; Sweeteners - stevia, erythritol, xylitol, monk fruit sugar. I use mostly stevia and erythritol. The latter is a sugar alcohol, but it doesn't spike blood sugar thanks to its zero glycemic indexes; Milk - consume full-fat coconut milk or almond milk; Flour - coconut or almond flour and almond meal; Oils - olive oil, avocado oil; Fats - butter or ghee.

What To Avoid

For you to stay on track with your Keto diet, there are certain foods that you need to say farewell to:

Sugar, honey, agave, soda, and sugary drinks, and fruit juices. Starchy vegetables such as potatoes, beans, legumes, peas, yams, and corn are usually packed with tons of carbs, so they must be avoided. However, sneaking some starch when your daily carb limit allows, is not exactly a sin. Flours - all-purpose, wheat, and rice. Dried fruits and fruit in general, except for berries. Grains — rice, wheat, and everything made from grains such as pasta or traditional bread are not allowed. No margarine, milk, refined oils, and fats such as corn oil, canola oil, vegetable oil, etc.

Keto Swaps

Just because you are not allowed to eat rice or pasta, doesn't mean that you have to sacrifice eating risotto or spaghetti. Well, sort of. For every forbidden item on the keto diet, there is a healthier replacement that will not contradict your dietary goal and will still taste amazing.

Here are the last keto swaps that you need to know to overcome the cravings quicker, and become a Keto chef:

Bread and Buns - Bread made from nut flour, mushroom caps, cucumber slices

Wraps and Tortillas - Wraps and tortillas made from nut flour, lettuce leaves, kale leaves

Pasta and Spaghetti - Spiralized veggies such as zoodles, spaghetti squash, etc.

Lasagna Noodles - Zucchini or eggplant slices

Rice - Cauliflower rice (ground in a food processor)

Mashed Potatoes - Mashed Cauliflower or other veggies

Hash Browns - Cauliflower or Spaghetti squash

Flour - Coconut flour, Hazelnut flour, Almond Flour

Breadcrumbs - Almond flour

Pizza Crust - Crust made with almond flour or cauliflower crust

French Fries - Carrot sticks, Turnip fries, Zucchini fries

Potato Chips - Zucchini chips, Kale chips

Croutons - Bacon bits, nuts, sunflower seeds, flax crackers

Getting Started With Your Keto Diet

Before starting the keto diet, take some time to research the foods on the allowed list and those restricted foods. Plan your meals ahead of time and shop accordingly, filling your kitchen with keto-friendly foods.

Healthy Snacks

To make it easier to stick to the keto diet, it's important to have healthy snacks. If you're on the keto diet with your partner, have keto-approved snacks on hand that you both enjoy. Approved snacks include:

• Hard-boiled eggs, cheese, and olives
• A handful of nuts and seeds
• Celery and red pepper sticks with guacamole and salsa
• No-sugar plain yogurt mixed with berries

Chapter 1. Breakfast Recipes

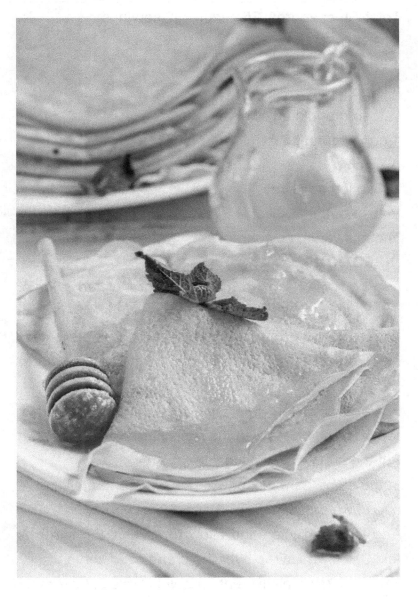

1 Lemon Crepes

Total Time: approx. 25 minutes |2 servings

INGREDIENTS:

1 cup almond milk, softened

3 large eggs

½ tbsp granulated swerve

1 cup almond flour

A pinch of salt

1 tbsp lemon juice

½ tbsp butter

¾ cup swerve, powdered

DIRECTIONS:

In a bowl, mix almond milk, eggs, granulated swerve, salt, and almond flour until well incorporated.

Grease a frying pan with cooking spray and set over medium heat; cook the crepes until the edges start to brown, about 2 minutes.

Flip and cook the other side for a further 2 minutes; repeat the process with the remaining batter.

Put the crepes on a plate.

In the same pan, mix powdered swerve, butter and ½ cup of water; simmer for 6 minutes as you stir.

Add in lemon juice and allow to sit until the syrup is thick. Pour the syrup over the crepes and serve.

NUTRITION: Cal 251; Fat 20g; Net Carbs 5.3g; Protein 7g

Total Time: approx. 40 minutes |4 servings

INGREDIENTS:

3 eggs

½ cup cottage cheese

1 tbsp coconut flour

1/3 cup Parmesan, grated

A pinch of xanthan gum

1 cup spinach

4 oz turkey bacon, cubed

4 oz mozzarella, shredded

1 garlic clove, minced

½ onion, chopped

2 tbsp butter

½ cup heavy cream

Fresh parsley, chopped

Salt and black pepper, to taste

DIRECTIONS:

In a bowl, combine cottage cheese, eggs, coconut flour, xanthan, and Parmesan cheese to obtain a crepe batter.

Grease a pan with cooking spray over medium heat, pour some of the batter, spread well into the pan, cook for 2 minutes, flip, and cook for 40 seconds more or until golden.

Do the same with the rest of the batter.

Stack all the crepes on a serving plate.

In the same pan, melt the butter and stir in the onion and garlic; sauté for 3 minutes, until tender.

Stir in the spinach and cook for 5 minutes.

Add in the turkey bacon, heavy cream, mozzarella cheese, pepper, and stir.

Cook for 2-3 minutes.

Fill each crepe with this mixture, roll up each one, and arrange on a serving plate.

Top with parsley.

NUTRITION: Cal 321; Fat 21g; Net Carbs 5.2g; Protein 26g

3 Bacon Quiche with Cheddar Cheese

Prep time: 5 minutes | Cook time: 12 minutes | Serves 2

INGREDIENTS:

3 large eggs

2 tablespoons heavy whipping cream

¼ teaspoon salt

4 slices cooked sugar-free bacon, crumbled

½ cup shredded mild Cheddar cheese

DIRECTIONS:

In a large bowl, whisk eggs, cream, and salt together until combined. Mix in bacon and Cheddar.

Pour mixture evenly into two ungreased 4-inch ramekins. Place into air fryer basket. Adjust the temperature to 320°F (160°C) and set the timer for 12 minutes. Quiche will be fluffy and set in the middle when done.

Let quiche cool in ramekins 5 minutes. Serve warm.

NUTRITION: Cal: 380 | fat: 28g | protein: 24g | carbs: 2g | net carbs: 2g | fiber: 0g

Total Time: approx. 25 minutes |4 servings

INGREDIENTS:

3 eggs

½ cup buttermilk

½ cup almond flour

½ tsp baking powder

1 tbsp swerve sugar

1 lemon, juiced

1 vanilla pod

2 tbsp unsalted butter

2 tbsp olive oil

3 tbsp sugar-free maple syrup

Blueberries to serve

Greek yogurt to serve

DIRECTIONS:

In a small bowl, whisk the buttermilk, lemon juice, and eggs.

In another bowl, mix the almond flour, baking powder, and swerve sugar.

Fold in the egg mixture and whisk until smooth.

Cut the vanilla pod open and scrape the beans into the flour mixture.

Stir to incorporate evenly.

In a skillet, melt a quarter each of the butter and olive oil and spoon in 2 tablespoons of the pancake mixture into the pan.

Cook for 4 minutes or until small bubbles appear.

Flip and cook for 2 minutes or until set and golden.

Repeat cooking until the batter finishes using the remaining butter and olive oil in the same proportions.

Plate the pancakes, drizzle with maple syrup, top with a generous dollop of yogurt, and scatter some blueberries on top.

NUTRITION: Cal 172; Net Carbs 1.6g; Fat 12g; Protein 7g

5 Ginger Pancakes

Total Time: approx. 15 minutes |2 servings

INGREDIENTS:

1 cup almond flour

1 tsp cinnamon powder

2 tbsp swerve brown sugar

¼ tsp baking soda

1 tsp ginger powder

1 egg

1 cup almond milk

2 tbsp olive oil

Lemon sauce

¼ cup stevia

½ tsp arrowroot starch

½ lemon, juiced and zested

2 tbsp butter

DIRECTIONS:

Combine together the almond flour, cinnamon powder, swerve brown sugar, baking soda, ginger powder, egg, almond milk, and olive oil in a mixing bowl.

Heat oil in a skillet over medium heat and spoon 2-3 tablespoons of the mixture into the skillet.

Cook the batter for 1 minute, flip it and cook the other side for another minute.

Remove the pancake onto a plate and repeat the cooking process until the batter is exhausted.

Mix the stevia and arrowroot starch in a medium saucepan.

Set the pan over medium heat and gradually stir 1 cup water until it thickens, about 1 minute.

Turn the heat off and add the butter, lemon juice, and lemon zest.

Stir the mixture until the butter melts.

Drizzle the sauce over the pancakes and serve them warm.

NUTRITION: Cal 343; Fat 25g; Net Carbs 6.1g; Protein 8g

Chapter 2. Snack & Appetizer Recipes

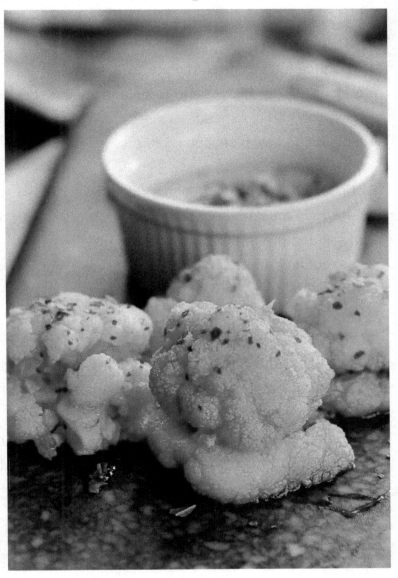

Prep time: 15 minutes | Cook time: 25 minutes | Serves 10

INGREDIENTS:

1½ pounds (680 g) ground chicken

8 ounces (227 g) Parmigiano-Reggiano cheese, grated

1 teaspoon garlic, minced

1 tablespoon Italian seasoning mix

1 egg, whisked

8 ounces (227 g) spinach, chopped

½ teaspoon mustard seeds

Sea salt and ground black pepper, to taste

½ teaspoon paprika

DIRECTIONS:

Mix the ingredients until everything is well incorporated.

Now, shape the meat mixture into 20 meatballs. Transfer your meatballs to a baking sheet and brush them with a nonstick cooking oil.

Bake in the preheated oven at 390ºF (199ºC) for about 25 minutes or until golden brown. Serve with cocktail sticks and enjoy!

NUTRITION:

calories: 210 | fat: 12.4g | protein: 19.4g | carbs: 4.5g | net carbs: 4.0g | fiber: 0.5g

Prep time: 10 minutes | Cook time: 20 minutes | Serves 6

INGREDIENTS:

6 eggs

1 tablespoon green tabasco

⅓ cup sugar-free mayonnaise

DIRECTIONS:

Place the eggs in a saucepan, and cover with salted water. Bring to a boil over medium heat. Boil for 8 minutes. Place the eggs in an ice bath and let cool for 10 minutes. Peel and slice them in. Whisk together the tabasco, mayonnaise, and salt in a small bowl. Spoon this mixture on top of every egg.

NUTRITION:

calories: 180 | fat: 17.0g | protein: 6.0g | carbs: 5.0g | net carbs: 5.0g | fiber: 0g

Prep time: 10 minutes | Cook time: 30 minutes | Serves 2

INGREDIENTS:

1½ cups cauliflower florets

1 tablespoon butter, softened

1 egg, whisked

Sea salt and ground black pepper, to taste

1 teaspoon Italian seasoning mix

½ cup Asiago cheese, grated

DIRECTIONS:

Pulse the cauliflower in your food processor; now, heat the butter in a nonstick skillet and cook the cauliflower until golden.

Add the remaining ingredients and blend together until well incorporated.

Form the mixture into balls and flatten them with the palm of your hand. Arrange on a tinfoil-lined baking pan.

Bake in the preheated oven at 400°F (205°C) for 25 to 30 minutes. Serve with homemade ketchup. Bon appétit!

NUTRITION:

calories: 235 | fat: 19.1g | protein: 12.4g | carbs: 4.4g | net carbs: 2.9g | fiber: 1.5g

Prep time: 15 minutes | Cook time: 30 minutes | Serves 8

INGREDIENTS:

1¼ cups Romano cheese, grated

½ cup Asiago cheese, grated

2 ripe tomatoes, peeled

½ teaspoon sea salt

½ teaspoon chili powder

1 teaspoon dried oregano

1 teaspoon dried basil

1 teaspoon dried parsley flakes

1 teaspoon garlic powder

DIRECTIONS:

Mix the cheese in a bowl. Place tablespoon-sized heaps of the mixture onto parchment lined baking pans.

Bake in the preheated oven at 380°F (193°C) approximately 7 minutes until beginning to brown around the edges.

Let them stand for about 15 minutes until crisp.

Meanwhile, purée the tomatoes in your food processor. Bring the puréed tomatoes to a simmer, add the remaining ingredients and cook for 30 minutes or until it has thickened and cooked through.

Serve the cheese crisps with the spicy tomato sauce on the side. Bon appétit!

NUTRITION: Cal.: 110 | fat: 7.5g | protein: 8.4g | carbs: 2.0g | net carbs: 1.6g | fiber: 0.4g

10 Caprese Sticks

Prep time: 10 minutes | Cook time: 0 minutes | Serves 8

INGREDIENTS:

2 tablespoons extra-virgin olive oil

2 tablespoons red wine vinegar

1 tablespoon Italian seasoning blend

8 pieces Prosciutto

8 pieces Soppressata

16 grape tomatoes

8 black olives, pitted

8 ounces (227 g) Mozzarella, cubed

2 tablespoons fresh basil leaves, chopped

1 red bell pepper, sliced

1 yellow bell pepper, sliced

Coarse sea salt, to taste

DIRECTIONS:

In a small mixing bowl, make the vinaigrette by whisking the oil, vinegar, and Italian seasoning blend. Set aside.

Slide the ingredients on the prepared skewers.

Arrange the sticks on serving platter. Season with salt to taste. Serve the vinaigrette on the side and enjoy!

NUTRITION:

calories: 142 | fat: 8.3g | protein: 12.8g | carbs: 3.2g | net carbs: 2.2g | fiber: 1.0g

Chapter 3. Poultry Recipes

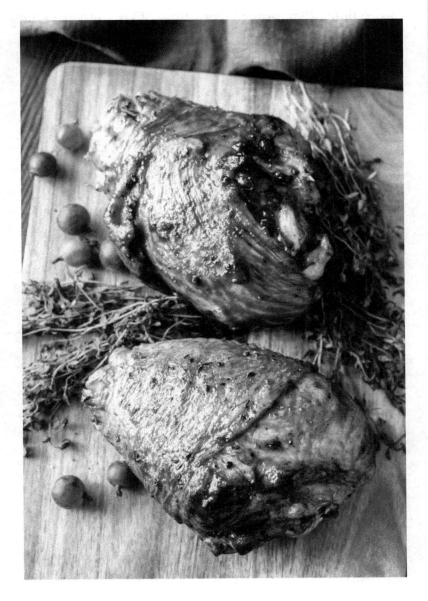

Prep time: 25 minutes | Cook time: 23 minutes | Serves 2

INGREDIENTS:

1 tablespoon red curry paste

½ teaspoon cayenne pepper

1½ tablespoons minced ginger

2 turkey drumsticks

¼ cup coconut milk

1 teaspoon kosher salt, or more to taste

⅓ teaspoon ground pepper, to more to taste

DIRECTIONS:

First of all, place turkey drumsticks with all ingredients in your refrigerator; let it marinate overnight.

Cook turkey drumsticks at 380ºF (193ºC) for 23 minutes; make sure to flip them over at half-time. Serve with the salad on the side.

NUTRITION: Cal: 298 | fat: 16g | protein: 12g | carbs: 25g | net carbs: 22g | fiber: 3g

Ready in about: 65 minutes | Serves: 6

INGREDIENTS:

2 medium lemons, sliced

3 chicken breasts, halved

Salt and black pepper to taste

¼ cup almond flour

3 tbsp olive oil

2 tbsp capers, rinsed

1 ¼ cups chicken vegetable broth

2 tbsp fresh parsley, chopped

1 tbsp butter

DIRECTIONS:

Preheat oven to 350ºF. Line a baking sheet with parchment paper. Lay the lemon slices on the baking sheet and drizzle with some olive oil. Roast for 25 minutes until the lemon rinds brown.

Cover the chicken with plastic wrap, place them on a flat surface, and gently pound with the rolling pin to flatten to about ½-inch thickness. Remove the plastic wraps and season with salt and pepper. Dredge the chicken in the almond flour on each side, and shake off any excess flour. Set aside.

Heat the remaining olive oil in a skillet over medium heat. Fry the chicken on both sides until golden brown, about 8 minutes. Pour in the vegetable broth and let it boil until it becomes thick in consistency, 12 minutes.

Stir in the capers, butter, and roasted lemons and simmer on low heat for 10 minutes. Turn the heat off. Pour the sauce over the chicken and garnish with parsley to serve.

NUTRITION: Cal 430, Fat 23g, Net Carbs 3g, Protein 33g

Ready in about: 60 minutes | Serves: 4

INGREDIENTS:

Chicken

4 chicken breasts

1 cup baby spinach

¼ cup goat cheese

¼ cup cheddar cheese, shredded

4 tbsp butter, melted

Salt and black pepper to taste

Tomato sauce

1 tbsp butter

1 shallot, chopped

2 garlic cloves, chopped

½ tbsp liquid stevia

2 tbsp tomato paste

14 oz canned crushed tomatoes

Salt and black pepper to taste

1 tsp dried basil

1 tsp dried oregano

Salad

2 cucumbers, spiralized

2 tbsp olive oil

1 tbsp white wine vinegar

DIRECTIONS:

Preheat oven to 400ºF. Place a pan over medium heat. Warm 2 tbsp of butter and sauté spinach until it shrinks. Season with salt and pepper. Transfer to a bowl containing goat cheese, stir, and set aside.

Cut the chicken breasts lengthwise and stuff with the cheese mixture. Set into a baking dish. On top, spread the cheddar cheese and add 2 tbsp of butter. Bake until cooked through for 25-30 minutes.

Warm 1 tbsp of the butter in a pan over medium heat. Add in garlic and shallot and cook for 3 minutes until soft. Stir in herbs, tomato paste, stevia, tomatoes, salt, and pepper and cook for 15 minutes.

Arrange the cucumbers on a serving platter, season with salt, pepper, olive oil, and vinegar. Top with the chicken and pour over the sauce. Serve.

NUTRITION: Cal: 453, Fat: 31g, Net Carbs: 6g, Protein: 43g

14. Creamy Stuffed Chicken with Parma Ham

Ready in about: 40 minutes | Serves: 4

INGREDIENTS:

4 chicken breasts

2 tbsp olive oil

2 cloves garlic, minced

2 shallots, finely chopped

1 tsp dried mixed herbs

8 slices Parma ham

4 oz cream cheese, softened

1 lemon, zested

Salt to taste

DIRECTIONS:

Preheat oven to 350°F. Heat the oil in a skillet over medium heat. Sauté garlic and shallots for 3 minutes. Stir the cream cheese, mixed herbs, salt, and lemon zest for 2 minutes. Remove and let cool.

Score a pocket in each chicken breast, fill the holes with the cheese mixture, and cover with the cut-out chicken. Wrap each breast with 2 ham slices and secure the ends with a toothpick. Lay the chicken parcels on a greased baking sheet. Bake for 20 minutes. Remove and let it rest for 4 minutes. Serve.

NUTRITION: Cal 485, Fat 35g, Net Carbs 2g, Protein 26g

Ready in about: 35 minutes + marinating time | Serves: 4

INGREDIENTS:

12 chicken wings, cut in half

1 tbsp turmeric

1 tbsp cumin

3 tbsp fresh ginger, grated

2 tbsp cilantro, chopped

½ tsp paprika

Salt and black pepper to taste

4 tbsp olive oil

Juice of ½ lime

2 tbsp fresh thyme, chopped

¾ cup cilantro, chopped

1 jalapeño pepper, chopped

DIRECTIONS:

In a bowl, stir 1 tbsp ginger, cumin, paprika, salt, 2 tbsp olive oil, black pepper, and turmeric. Place in the chicken wings pieces and toss to coat. Marinate in the fridge for 20 minutes. Remove before grilling.

Heat the grill, place in the marinated wings, and cook for 25 minutes, turning from time to time. Remove and set to a serving plate. Blitz thyme, remaining ginger, salt, jalapeno, black pepper, lime juice, cilantro, remaining olive oil, and 1 tbsp water in a blender. Drizzle the chicken wings with the sauce and serve.

NUTRITION: Cal 243, Fat 15g, Net Carbs 3.5g, Protein 22g

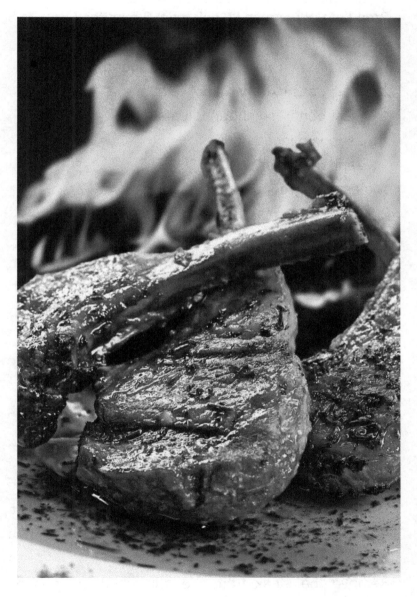

16 Balsamic Skirt Steak

Prep time: 2 minutes | Cook time: 6 minutes | Serves 6

INGREDIENTS:

¼ cup balsamic vinegar (no sugar added)

2 tablespoons extra-virgin olive oil

1 tablespoon fresh chopped parsley

1 teaspoon minced garlic

1 teaspoon kosher salt

¼ teaspoon ground black pepper

2 pounds (907 g) skirt steak, trimmed of fat

DIRECTIONS:

In a medium-sized bowl, whisk together the vinegar, olive oil, parsley, garlic, salt, and pepper. Add the skirt steak and flip to ensure that the entire surface is covered in marinade. Cover with plastic wrap and marinate in the refrigerator for at least 2 hours, or up to 24 hours.

Take the bowl out of the refrigerator and let the steak and marinade come to room temperature. Meanwhile, preheat a grill to high heat.

Remove the steak from the marinade (reserve the marinade) and place on the grill over direct high heat. Grill for 3 minutes per side for medium (recommended) or 5 minutes per side for well-done.

Remove the steak from the grill when the desired doneness is reached and let rest for 10 minutes before slicing. Meanwhile, place the reserved marinade in the microwave and cook on high for 3 minutes, or until boiling. Stir and set aside; you will use the boiled marinade as a sauce for the steak.

Slice the steak, being sure to cut against the grain for best results. Serve with the sauce.

NUTRITION:

calories: 355 | fat: 25.1g | protein: 30.9g | carbs: 0g | net carbs: 0g | fiber: 0g

Ready in about: 30 minutes | Serves: 4

Ingredients

2 eggplants

2 tbsp olive oil

1 ½ lb ground beef

1 medium red onion, chopped

1 roasted red pepper, chopped

Pink salt and black pepper to taste

1 cup yellow cheddar cheese, grated

2 tbsp dill, chopped

DIRECTIONS:

Preheat oven to 350ºF. Lay the eggplants on a flat surface, trim off the ends, and cut in half lengthwise. Scoop out the pulp from each half to make shells. Chop the pulp. Heat oil in a skillet over medium heat. Add the ground beef, red onion, pimiento, and eggplant pulp and season with salt and pepper.

Cook for 6 minutes while stirring to break up lumps until beef is no longer pink. Spoon the beef into the eggplant shells and sprinkle with cheddar cheese. Place on a greased baking sheet and cook to melt the cheese for 15 minutes until eggplant is tender. Serve warm topped with dill.

NUTRITION: Cal 574, Fat 27.5g, Net Carbs 9.8g, Protein 61,8g

Ready in about: 35 minutes + marinating time | Serves: 4

Ingredients

4 tbsp sugar-free BBQ sauce + extra for serving

2 tbsp erythritol

Pink salt and black pepper to taste

2 tbsp olive oil

2 tsp chipotle powder

1 tsp garlic powder

1 lb beef spare ribs

DIRECTIONS:

Mix the erythritol, salt, pepper, oil, chipotle, and garlic powder. Brush on the meaty sides of the ribs and wrap in foil. Sit for 30 minutes to marinate.

Preheat oven to 400°F. Place wrapped ribs on a baking sheet and cook for 40 minutes until cooked through. Remove ribs and aluminum foil, brush with BBQ sauce, and brown under the broiler for 10 minutes on both sides. Slice and serve with extra BBQ sauce and lettuce tomato salad.

NUTRITION: Cal 395, Fat 33g, Net Carbs 3g, Protein 21g

Prep time: 15 minutes | Cook time: 35 minutes | Serves 6

INGREDIENTS:

5 pounds (2.3 kg) beef rib roast, on the bone

3 heads garlic, cut in half

3 tablespoons olive oil

6 shallots, peeled and halved

2 lemons, zested and juiced

3 tablespoons mustard seeds

3 tablespoons Swerve

Salt and black pepper to taste

3 tablespoons thyme leaves

DIRECTIONS:

Preheat oven to 450ºF (235ºC). Place garlic heads and shallots in a roasting dish, toss with olive oil, and bake for 15 minutes. Pour lemon juice on them. Score shallow crisscrosses patterns on the meat and set aside.

Mix Swerve, mustard seeds, thyme, salt, pepper, and lemon zest to make a rub; and apply it all over the beef. Place the beef on the shallots and garlic; cook in the oven for 15 minutes. Reduce the heat to 400ºF (205ºC), cover the dish with foil, and continue cooking for 5 minutes.

Once ready, remove the dish, and let sit covered for 15 minutes before slicing.

NUTRITION:

calories: 555 | fat: 38.5g | protein: 58.3g | carbs: 7.7g | net carbs: 2.4g | fiber: 5.3g

20 Grilled Sirloin Steak with Sauce Diane

Ready in about: 25 minutes | Serves: 6

INGREDIENTS:

Sirloin steak

1 ½ lb sirloin steak

Salt and black pepper to taste

1 tsp olive oil

Sauce Diane

1 tbsp olive oil

1 clove garlic, minced

1 cup sliced porcini mushrooms

1 small onion, finely diced

2 tbsp butter

1 tbsp Dijon mustard

2 tbsp Worcestershire sauce

¼ cup whiskey

2 cups heavy cream

DIRECTIONS:

Put a grill pan over high heat and as it heats, brush the steak with oil, sprinkle with salt and pepper, and rub the seasoning into the meat with your hands. Cook the steak in the pan for 4 minutes on each side for medium-rare and transfer to a chopping board to rest for 4 minutes before slicing. Reserve the juice.

Heat the oil in a frying pan over medium heat and sauté the onion for 3 minutes. Add the butter, garlic, and mushrooms, and cook for 2 minutes. Add the Worcestershire sauce, the reserved juice, and mustard. Stir and cook for 1 minute. Pour in the whiskey and cook further 1 minute until the sauce reduces by half. Swirl the pan and add the cream. Let it simmer to thicken for about 3 minutes. Adjust the taste with salt and pepper. Spoon the sauce over the steaks slices and serve with celeriac mash.

NUTRITION: Cal 434, Fat 17g, Net Carbs 2.9g, Protein 36g

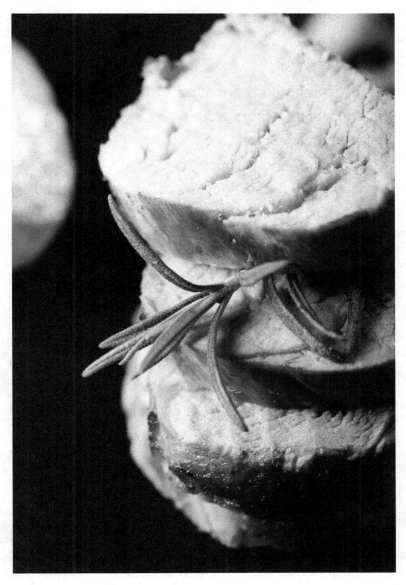

Prep time: 10 minutes | Cook time: 35 minutes |
Serves 4

INGREDIENTS:

½ teaspoon ground coriander

2 cups beef vegetable broth

½ teaspoon cocoa powder

1 teaspoon Ancho chili powder

1 pound (454 g) pork shoulder, boneless, chopped

DIRECTIONS:

Put ground coriander, beef vegetable broth, and cocoa powder in the Instant Pot.

Stir the mixture until the beef vegetable broth turns color into chocolate.

Add the Ancho chili powder and pork shoulder.

Close the lid. Select Meat/Stew mode and set cooking time for 35 minutes on High Pressure.

When the timer beeps, use a natural pressure release for 15 minutes, then release any remaining pressure. Open the lid.

Serve warm.

NUTRITION:

calories: 351 | fat: 25.0g | protein: 28.9g | carbs: 0.6g | net carbs: 0.5g | fiber: 0.1g

22 Pork Fillet and Tomato Salad

Prep time: 10 minutes | Cook time: 15 minutes | Serves 4

INGREDIENTS:

10 ounces (283 g) pork fillet

½ teaspoon chicken seasonings

1 tablespoon olive oil

⅓ cup water

1 tomato, chopped

⅓ cup black olives, sliced

1 cup lettuce, chopped

DIRECTIONS:

Slice the pork fillet and sprinkle with chicken seasonings.

Place the fillet slices in the Instant Pot, then add olive oil and cook on Sauté mode for 5 minutes. Stir constantly.

When the meat is light browned, add water and close the lid.

Select Meat/Stew mode and set cooking time for 10 minutes on High Pressure.

Meanwhile, in the salad bowl, mix the tomato, black olives, and lettuce.

Top the salad with the cooked pork slices. Toss and serve.

NUTRITION: calories: 213 | fat: 13.8g | protein: 20.0g | carbs: 1.7g | net carbs: 1.1g | fiber: 0.6g

Ready in about: 23 minutes | Serves: 4

INGREDIENTS:

2 tbsp ghee

2 lb pork loin, cut into strips

Pink salt to taste

2 tsp ginger-garlic paste

¼ cup chicken vegetable broth

5 tbsp peanut butter, softened

2 cups mixed stir-fry vegetables

½ tsp chili pepper

DIRECTIONS:

Melt the ghee in a wok over high heat. Rub the pork with salt, chili pepper, and ginger-garlic paste. Place it into the wok and cook for 6 minutes until no longer pink. Mix peanut butter and vegetable broth until smooth.

Pour in the wok and stir for 6 minutes. Add in the mixed veggies and simmer for 5 minutes. Adjust the taste with salt and black pepper and spoon the stir-fry to a side of cilantro cauli rice.

NUTRITION: Cal 571, Fat 49g, Net Carbs 1g, Protein 22.5g

Ready in about: 20 minutes + marinating time | Serves: 4

NUTRITION: Cal 315, Fat 18g, Net Carbs 2.3g, Protein 36g

Ingredients

¼ cup lime juice

4 pork chops

2 tbsp coconut oil, melted

2 garlic cloves, minced

½ tsp chili powder

1 tsp ground cinnamon

Salt and black pepper to taste

½ tsp hot pepper sauce

4 dill pickles, cut into spears

DIRECTIONS:

In a bowl, combine the lime juice with coconut oil, salt, hot pepper sauce, black pepper, cinnamon, garlic, and chili powder. Place in the pork chops, toss to coat, and refrigerate for 4 hours.

Arrange the pork on the preheated grill over medium heat and cook for 7 minutes. Turn, add in the dill pickles, and cook for another 7 minutes. Split among serving plates and serve.

Ready in about: 35 minutes | Serves: 4

NUTRITION: Cal 495, Fat 29g, Net Carbs 2.7g, Protein 36.5g

Ingredients

1 lb ground pork

1 large yellow squash, thinly sliced

Salt and black pepper to taste

1 clove garlic, minced

4 green onions, chopped

1 cup chopped cremini mushrooms

1 (15 oz) can diced tomatoes

½ cup pork rinds, crushed

2 tbsp fresh parsley, chopped

1 cup cottage cheese, crumbled

1 cup Mexican cheese blend

3 tbsp olive oil

DIRECTIONS:

Preheat oven to 370ºF. Heat the olive oil in a skillet over medium heat. Add in the pork, season with salt and black pepper, and cook for 3 minutes or until no longer pink. Stir occasionally while breaking any lumps apart. Add the garlic, half of the green onions, mushrooms, and 2 tablespoons of pork rinds.

Cook for 3 minutes. Stir in the tomatoes and ⅓ cup water. Cook for 3 minutes. Remove the pan. Mix the parsley, cottage cheese, and Mexican cheese blend in a bowl. Sprinkle the bottom of a baking dish with some pork rinds, top with half of the squash, and season with salt. Top with 2/3 of the pork mixture and 2/3 of the cheese mixture. Repeat the layering process a second time to exhaust the ingredients.

Cover the baking dish with foil and bake for 20 minutes. After, remove the foil and brown the top of the casserole with the oven's broiler side for 2 minutes. Remove the dish when ready and serve warm.

Chapter 6. Fish and Seafood

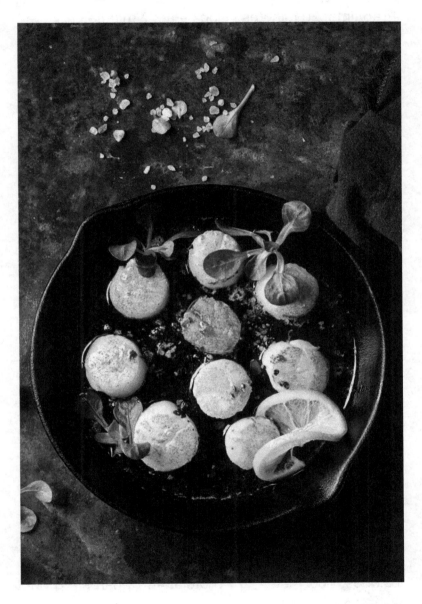

26 Cheese Shrimp

Prep time: 20 minutes | Cook time: 7 minutes | Serves 4

INGREDIENTS:

2 egg whites

½ cup coconut flour

1 cup Parmigiano-Reggiano, grated

½ teaspoon celery seeds

½ teaspoon porcini powder

½ teaspoon onion powder

1 teaspoon garlic powder

½ teaspoon dried rosemary

½ teaspoon sea salt

½ teaspoon ground black pepper

1½ pounds (680g) shrimp, deveined

DIRECTIONS:

Whisk the egg with coconut flour and Parmigiano-Reggiano. Add in seasonings and mix to combine well. Dip your shrimp in the batter. Roll until they are covered on all sides.

Cook in the preheated Air Fryer at 390°F (199°C) for 5 to 7 minutes or until golden brown. Work in batches. Serve with lemon wedges if desired.

NUTRITION:

calories: 300 | fat: 11g | protein: 44g | carbs: 7g | net carbs: 6g | fiber: 1g

Prep time: 10 minutes | Cook time: 6 minutes | Serves 4

INGREDIENTS:

12 ounces (340 g) scallops

1 tablespoon dried rosemary

½ teaspoon Pink salt

1 tablespoon avocado oil

DIRECTIONS:

Sprinkle scallops with dried rosemary, Pink salt, and avocado oil.

Then put the scallops in the air fryer basket in one layer and cook at 400°F (205°C) for 6 minutes.

NUTRITION:

calories: 82 | fat: 1g | protein: 14g | carbs: 3g | net carbs: 2g | fiber: 1g

Prep time: 5 minutes | Cook time: 10 minutes | Serves 4

INGREDIENTS:

1 tablespoon butter

1 teaspoon fresh grated ginger

2 garlic cloves, minced

2 tablespoon chopped green onions

1 pound (454 g) swai fish fillets

½ cup port wine

1 teaspoon parsley flakes

½ tablespoon lemon juice

½ teaspoon chili flakes

½ teaspoon cayenne pepper

½ teaspoon fennel seeds

¼ teaspoon ground bay leaf

Coarse sea salt and ground black pepper, to taste

DIRECTIONS:

Set your Instant Pot to Sauté and melt the butter.

Cook the ginger, garlic, and green onions for 2 minutes until softened. Add the remaining ingredients and gently stir to incorporate.

Lock the lid. Select the Manual mode and set the cooking time for 6 minutes at Low Pressure.

When the timer beeps, perform a quick pressure release. Carefully remove the lid.

Serve warm.

NUTRITION:

calories: 112 | fat: 3.5g | protein: 17.8g | carbs: 1.7g | net carbs: 1.3g | fiber: 0.4g

29 Red Cabbage Tilapia Bowl

Ready in about: 20 minutes | Serves: 4

INGREDIENTS:

2 cups cauli rice

2 tsp ghee

4 tilapia fillets, cut into cubes

Salt and chili pepper to taste

¼ head red cabbage, shredded

1 ripe avocado, pitted and chopped

DIRECTIONS:

Sprinkle cauli rice in a bowl with a little water and microwave for 3 minutes. Fluff after with a fork and set aside. Melt ghee in a skillet over medium heat, rub the tilapia with the taco seasoning, salt, and chili pepper and fry until brown on all sides, about 8 minutes. Transfer to a plate and set aside. Share the cauli rice, cabbage, fish, and avocado in 4 serving bowls. Serve with chipotle lime sour cream dressing.

NUTRITION: Cal 269, Fat 23.4g, Net Carbs 4g, Protein 16.5g

Ready in about: 10 minutes | Serves: 2

INGREDIENTS:

4 cups zoodles (zucchini spirals)

2 oz cubed bacon

4 oz canned sardines, chopped

½ cup canned tomatoes, chopped

1 tbsp capers

1 garlic clove, minced

DIRECTIONS:

Pour some of the sardine oil in a pan over medium heat. Add the garlic and sauté for 1 minute. Stir in bacon and cook for 2 more minutes. Pour in the tomatoes and simmer for 5 minutes. Add zoodles and sardines and cook for 3 minutes. Transfer to a serving plate and top with capers. Serve.

NUTRITION: Cal 355, Fat: 31g, Net Carbs: 6g, Protein: 20g

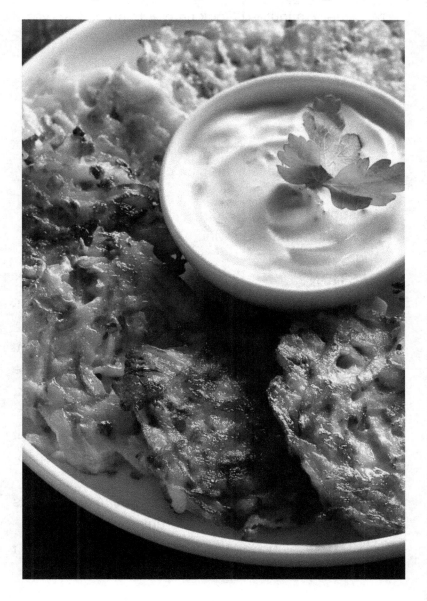

Prep time: 7 minutes | Cook time: 8 minutes | Serves 3

INGREDIENTS:

½ pound (227 g) fresh cauliflower

1 tablespoon sesame oil

½ cup leeks, chopped

1 garlic, pressed

Sea salt and freshly ground black pepper, to taste

½ teaspoon Chinese five-spice powder

1 teaspoon oyster sauce

½ teaspoon light soy sauce

1 tablespoon Shaoxing wine

3 eggs

DIRECTIONS:

Pulse the cauliflower in a food processor until it resembles rice.

Heat the sesame oil in a pan over medium-high heat; sauté the leeks and garlic for 2 to 3 minutes. Add the prepared cauliflower rice to the pan, along with salt, black pepper, and Chinese five-spice powder.

Next, add oyster sauce, soy sauce, and wine. Let it cook, stirring occasionally, until the cauliflower is crisp-tender, about 5 minutes.

Then, add the eggs to the pan; stir until everything is well combined. Serve warm and enjoy!

NUTRITION: calories: 132 | fat: 8.8g | protein: 7.2g | carbs: 6.2g | net carbs: 4.4g | fiber: 1.8g

Prep time: 5 minutes | Cook time: 10 minutes | Serves 3

INGREDIENTS:

2 tablespoons olive oil

½ shallot, diced

3 cloves garlic, chopped

12 ounces (340 g) brown mushrooms, thinly sliced

2 cups tomato sauce

DIRECTIONS:

Heat the olive oil in a stockpot over medium-high heat. Then, sauté the shallot for about 3 minutes until tender and fragrant.

Now, stir in the garlic and mushrooms and cook them for 1 minute more until aromatic.

Fold in the tomato sauce and bring to a boil; turn the heat to medium-low, cover, and continue to simmer for 5 to 6 minutes.

Salt to taste and serve over cauliflower rice if desired. Enjoy!

NUTRITION:

calories: 137 | fat: 9.3g | protein: 3.4g | carbs: 7.1g | net carbs: 5.3g | fiber: 1.8g

33 Zucchini Fritters

Prep time: 10 minutes | Cook time: 5 minutes | Serves 6

INGREDIENTS:

1 pound (454 g) zucchini, grated and drained

1 egg

1 teaspoon fresh Italian parsley

½ cup almond meal

½ cup goat cheese, crumbled

Sea salt and ground black pepper, to taste

½ teaspoon red pepper flakes, crushed

2 tablespoons olive oil

DIRECTIONS:

Mix all ingredients, except for the olive oil, in a large bowl. Let it sit in your refrigerator for 30 minutes.

Heat the oil in a non-stick frying pan over medium heat; scoop the heaped tablespoons of the zucchini mixture into the hot oil.

Cook for 3 to 4 minutes; then, gently flip the fritters over and cook on the other side. Cook in a couple of batches.

Transfer to a paper towel to soak up any excess grease. Serve and enjoy!

NUTRITION:

calories: 110 | fat: 8.8g | protein: 5.8g | carbs: 3.2g | net carbs: 2.2g | fiber: 1.0g

Prep time: 15 minutes | Cook time: 50 to 60 minutes | Serves 4

INGREDIENTS:

½ pound (227 g) spaghetti squash, halved, scoop out seeds

1 teaspoon olive oil

½ cup Mozzarella cheese, shredded

½ cup cream cheese

½ cup full-fat Greek yogurt

2 eggs

1 garlic clove, minced

½ teaspoon cumin

½ teaspoon basil ½ teaspoon mint

Sea salt and ground black pepper, to taste

DIRECTIONS:

Place the squash halves in a baking pan; drizzle the insides of each squash half with olive oil.

Bake in the preheated oven at 370ºF (188ºC) for 45 to 50 minutes or until the interiors are easily pierced through with a fork

Now, scrape out the spaghetti squash "noodles" from the skin in a mixing bowl. Add the remaining ingredients and mix to combine well.

Carefully fill each of the squash half with the cheese mixture. Bake at 350ºF (180ºC) for 5 to 10 minutes, until the cheese is bubbling and golden brown. Bon appétit!

NUTRITION:

calories: 220 | fat: 17.6g | protein: 9.0g | carbs: 6.8g | net carbs: 5.9g | fiber: 0.9g

Prep time: 20 minutes | Cook time: 40 minutes | Serves 6

INGREDIENTS:

1 (¾-pound / 340-g) eggplant, cut into ½-inch slices

1 tablespoon olive oil

1 tablespoon butter, melted

8 ounces (227 g) kale leaves, torn into pieces

14 ounces (397 g) garlic-and-tomato pasta sauce, without sugar

⅓ cup cream cheese

1 cup Asiago cheese, shredded

½ cup Gorgonzola cheese, grated

2 tablespoons ketchup, without sugar

1 teaspoon hot pepper

1 teaspoon basil

1 teaspoon oregano

½ teaspoon rosemary

DIRECTIONS:

Place the eggplant slices in a colander and sprinkle them with salt. Allow it to sit for 2 hours. Wipe the eggplant slices with paper towels.

Brush the eggplant slices with olive oil; cook in a cast-iron grill pan until nicely browned on both sides, about 5 minutes.

Melt the butter in a pan over medium flame. Now, cook the kale leaves until wilted. In a mixing bowl, combine the three types of cheese.

Transfer the grilled eggplant slices to a lightly greased baking dish. Top with the kale. Then, add a layer of ½ of cheese blend.

Pour the tomato sauce over the cheese layer. Top with the remaining cheese mixture. Sprinkle with seasoning. Bake in the preheated oven at 350ºF (180ºC) until cheese is bubbling and golden brown, about 35 minutes. Bon appétit!

NUTRITION:

calories: 231 | fat: 18.6g | protein: 10.5g | carbs: 6.7g | net carbs: 4.3g | fiber: 2.4g

Chapter 7. Salad Recipes

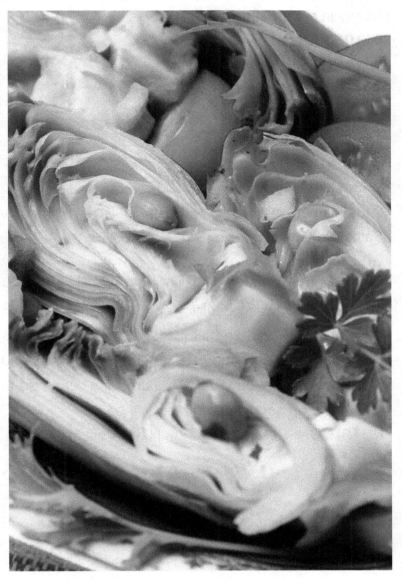

Ready in about: 30 minutes | Serves: 6

INGREDIENTS:

1 cauliflower head, florets only

1 lb medium shrimp, peeled

¼ cup + 1 tbsp olive oil

1 avocado, chopped

2 tbsp fresh dill, chopped

¼ cup lemon juice

2 tbsp lemon zest

Salt and black pepper to taste

DIRECTIONS:

Heat 1 tbsp olive oil in a skillet and cook shrimp for 8 minutes. Microwave cauliflower for 5 minutes. Place shrimp, cauliflower, and avocado in a bowl. Whisk the remaining olive oil, lemon zest, juice, dill, and salt, and pepper in another bowl. Pour the dressing over, toss to combine, and serve immediately.

NUTRITION: Cal 214, Fat: 17g, Net Carbs: 5g, Protein: 15g

37 Broccoli Slaw Salad with Mustard Vinaigrette

Ready in about: 10 minutes | Serves: 6

INGREDIENTS:

½ tsp granulated swerve sugar

1 tbsp Dijon mustard

2 tbsp olive oil

4 cups broccoli slaw

⅓ cup mayonnaise

1 tsp celery seeds

2 tbsp slivered almonds

1 ½ tbsp apple cider vinegar

Salt to taste

DIRECTIONS:

In a bowl, place the mayonnaise, Dijon mustard, swerve sugar, olive oil, celery seeds, vinegar, and salt and whisk until well combined. Place broccoli slaw in a large salad bowl. Pour the vinaigrette over. Toss to coat. Sprinkle with the slivered almonds and serve immediately.

NUTRITION: Cal 110, Fat: 10g, Net Carbs: 2g, Protein: 3g

38 Pork Burger Salad with Yellow Cheddar

Ready in about: 25 minutes | Serves: 4

INGREDIENTS:

½ lb ground pork

Salt and black pepper to taste

2 tbsp olive oil

2 hearts romaine lettuce, torn

2 firm tomatoes, sliced

¼ red onion, sliced

3 oz yellow cheddar cheese, grated

2 tbsp butter

DIRECTIONS:

Season the pork with salt and black pepper, mix, and make medium-sized patties out of them. Heat the butter in a skillet over medium heat and fry the patties on both sides for 10 minutes until browned and cook within. Transfer to a wire rack to drain oil. When cooled, cut into quarters.

Mix the lettuce, tomatoes, and red onion in a salad bowl, season with olive oil and salt. Toss and add the pork on top. Top with the cheese and serve.

NUTRITION: Cal 310, Fat 23g, Net Carbs 2g, Protein 22g

39 Warm Baby Artichoke Salad

Ready in about: 30 minutes | Serves: 4

INGREDIENTS:

6 baby artichokes

6 cups water

1 tbsp lemon juice

¼ cup cherry peppers, halved

¼ cup pitted olives, sliced

¼ cup olive oil

¼ tsp lemon zest

2 tsp balsamic vinegar, sugar-free

1 tbsp chopped dill

Salt and black pepper to taste

1 tbsp capers

¼ tsp caper brine

DIRECTIONS:

Combine the water and salt in a pot over medium heat. Trim and halve the artichokes. Add them to the pot and bring to a boil. Lower the heat and let simmer for 20 minutes until tender.

Combine the rest of the ingredients, except for the olives in a bowl. Drain and place the artichokes on a serving plate. Pour the prepared mixture over; toss to combine well. Serve topped with the olives.

NUTRITION: Cal 170, Fat: 13g, Net Carbs: 5g, Protein: 1g

Ready in about: 40 minutes | Serves: 4

INGREDIENTS:

2 turnips, cut into wedges

1 tsp olive oil

1 cup baby spinach, chopped

3 radishes, sliced

3 turkey bacon slices

4 tbsp sour cream

2 tsp mustard seeds

1 tsp Dijon mustard

1 tbsp red wine vinegar

Salt and black pepper to taste

1 tbsp chopped chives

DIRECTIONS:

Preheat oven to 400°F. Line a baking sheet with parchment paper, toss the turnips with salt and black pepper, drizzle with the olive oil, and bake for 25 minutes, turning halfway. Let cool.

Spread the baby spinach in the bottom of a salad bowl and top with the radishes. Remove the turnips to the salad bowl. Fry the bacon in a skillet over medium heat until crispy, about 5 minutes.

Mix sour cream, mustard seeds, mustard, vinegar, and salt with the bacon. Add a little water to deglaze the bottom of the skillet. Pour the bacon mixture over the vegetables, scatter the chives over it. Serve.

NUTRITION: Cal 193, Fat 18.3g, Net Carbs 3.1g, Protein 9.5g

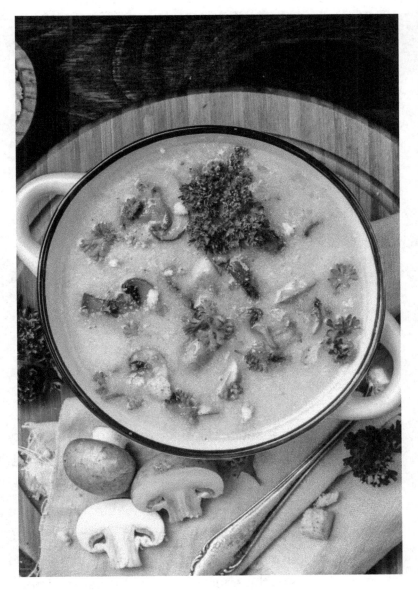

Total Time: approx. 25 minutes|4 servings

INGREDIENTS:

1 tbsp olive oil

6 slices bacon, chopped

1 tbsp butter

1 small white onion, chopped

3 garlic cloves, minced

2 tbsp finely chopped thyme

1 tbsp chopped fresh tarragon

1 tbsp chopped fresh oregano

2 cups cubed parsnips

3 ½ cups vegetable broth

Salt and black pepper to taste

1 cup almond milk

1 cup grated cheddar cheese

2 tbsp chopped scallions

DIRECTIONS:

Heat olive oil in a saucepan over medium heat and fry bacon until browned and crunchy, 5 minutes; set aside. Melt butter in the saucepan and sauté onion, garlic, thyme, tarragon, and oregano for 3 minutes. Add in the parsnips, season with salt and pepper, and cook for 15 minutes until the parsnips soften. Using an immersion blender, process the soup until smooth. Stir in almond milk and cheddar cheese and simmer with continuous stirring until the cheese melts. Top with bacon and scallions and serve.

NUTRITION: Cal 775; Net Carbs 6.5g; Fat 57g, Protein 18g

Total Time: approx. 25 minutes|4 servings

INGREDIENTS:

4 cups vegetable stock

1 cup pearl onions, halved

3 cups green beans, chopped

2 cups asparagus, chopped

2 cups baby spinach

1 tbsp garlic powder

Salt and white pepper to taste

2 cups grated Parmesan

DIRECTIONS:

Pour vegetable broth into a pot over medium heat and add pearl onions, green beans, and asparagus. Season with garlic powder, salt and white pepper and cook for 10 minutes. Stir in spinach and allow slight wilting. Top with Parmesan cheese and serve.

NUTRITION: Cal 196; Net Carbs 4.3g; Fat 12g, Protein 2.5g

Total Time: approx. 30 minutes|4 servings

INGREDIENTS:

12 oz wild mushrooms, chopped

¼ cup butter

5 oz crème fraiche

2 tsp fresh thyme, chopped

2 garlic cloves, minced

4 cups chicken broth

Salt and black pepper to taste

DIRECTIONS:

Melt butter in a large pot over medium heat. Add and sauté garlic for 1 minute until tender. Add in wild mushrooms, season with salt and pepper, and cook for 5 minutes. Pour the chicken broth over and bring to a boil. Reduce the heat and simmer for 10 minutes. Blitz with a hand blender until smooth. Stir in crème fraiche. Serve topped with thyme.

NUTRITION: Cal 281; Net Carbs 5.8g; Fat 25g, Protein 6g

Total Time: approx. 30 minutes |4 servings

INGREDIENTS:

½ lb chicken breasts, chopped

3 tbsp butter, melted

4 cups chicken broth

4 tbsp chopped cilantro

⅓ cup buffalo sauce

4 oz cream cheese

DIRECTIONS:

Blend butter, buffalo sauce, and cream cheese in a food processor until uniform and smooth. Transfer to a pot. Add the chicken to the pot, pour in the broth and cook for 20 minutes. Serve garnished with cilantro.

NUTRITION: Cal 406; Net Carbs 5g; Fat 29.5g, Protein 26g

Total Time: approx. 25 minutes|4 servings

INGREDIENTS:

1 cup cremini mushrooms, sliced and pre-cooked

1 tbsp olive oil

1 garlic clove, minced

1 white onion, finely chopped

1 tsp ginger puree

1 cup vegetable stock

2 turnips, peeled and chopped

Salt and black pepper to taste

1 cup feta cheese, crumbled

2 cups almond milk

1 tbsp chopped basil

Finely chopped parsley

Chopped walnuts for topping

DIRECTIONS:

Heat olive oil in a saucepan over medium heat and sauté garlic, onion, and ginger puree until fragrant and soft, about 3 minutes. Pour in vegetable stock, turnips and season with salt and pepper; cook for 6 minutes. Use an immersion blender to puree the ingredients until smooth. Stir in mushrooms and simmer covered for 7 minutes. Add in almond milk and heat for 2 minutes. Stir in basil and parsley and sprinkle with feta cheese. Serve warm.

NUTRITION: Cal 923; Net Carbs 7.4g; Fat 8.5g, Protein 23g

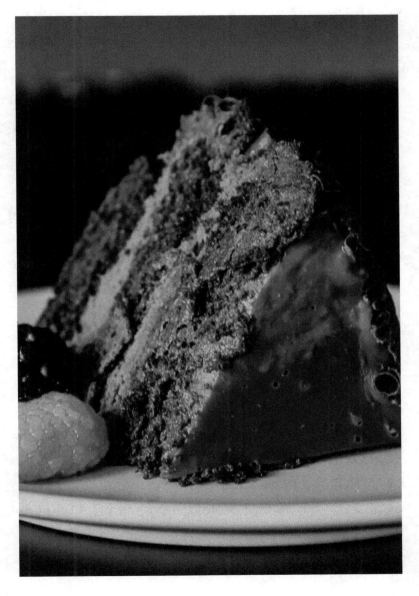

46 Strawberries Coated with Chocolate Chips

Prep time: 10 minutes | Cook time: 5 minutes | Makes 15

INGREDIENTS:

5 ounces (142 g) sugar-free dark chocolate chips

1 tablespoon vegetable shortening or lard

15 medium whole strawberries, fresh or frozen

DIRECTIONS:

Line the baking sheet with parchment paper and set aside.

In the microwave-safe bowl, combine the chocolate and shortening. Melt in the microwave in 30-second intervals, stirring in between.

Dip the strawberries into the melted chocolate mixture and place them on the prepared baking sheet.

Put the strawberries in the freezer for 10 to 15 minutes to set before serving.

Store leftovers in an airtight container in the refrigerator for up to 3 days.

NUTRITION: (3 Strawberries)

Cal: 216 | fat: 18.0g | protein: 4.0g | carbs: 11.0g | net carbs: 6.0g | fiber: 5.0g

47 Cream Cheese Chocolate Cake

Prep time: 15 minutes | Cook time: 20 minutes | Serves 10

INGREDIENTS:

1 stick butter, room temperature

⅓ cup full-fat milk

2 eggs

½ cup walnut meal

⅓ cup flaxseed meal

⅓ cup coconut flour

1 teaspoon baking powder

2 teaspoons liquid stevia

¼ teaspoon ground star anise

¼ teaspoon cinnamon

¼ teaspoon ground cloves

A pinch of flaky salt

2 tablespoons cocoa powder

1 teaspoon rum extract

Cream Cheese Frosting:

⅓ cup butter, room temperature

6 ounces (170 g) cream cheese, softened

½ cup Xylitol

½ teaspoon pure caramel extract

DIRECTIONS:

Cream the butter and milk with an electric mixer; slowly, fold in the eggs and beat again to combine well.

In another bowl, mix all types of flours with the baking powder, stevia, spices, cocoa powder, and rum extract. Now, stir this dry mixture into the wet mixture; mix again until everything is well incorporated.

Press the batter into a parchment-lined baking pan. Bake in the preheated oven at 400°F (205°C) for 18 minutes.

Meanwhile, whip the butter and cream cheese with an electric mixer.

Add in the Xylitol and caramel extract; continue to beat until the sweetener is well dissolved and the frosting is creamy.

Frost your cake and serve well-chilled. Bon appétit!

NUTRITION:

Cal: 293 | fat: 29.2g | protein: 5.2g | carbs: 5.4g | net carbs: 3.1g | fiber: 2.3g

Prep time: 10 minutes | Cook time: 0 minutes | Serves 6

INGREDIENTS:

1 (13.5-ounce / 383-g) can coconut cream, chilled overnight

3 tablespoons granulated erythritol–monk fruit blend; less sweet: 2 tablespoons

2 tablespoons unsweetened cocoa powder, plus more for dusting

1 teaspoon instant espresso powder

¼ teaspoon salt

DIRECTIONS:

Put the large metal bowl in the freezer to chill for at least 1 hour.

In the chilled large bowl, using an electric mixer on high, combine the coconut cream (adding it by the spoonful and reserving the water that has separated), erythritol–monk fruit blend, the cocoa powder, espresso powder, and salt and beat for 3 to 5 minutes, until stiff peaks form, stopping and scraping the bowl once or twice, as needed. If the consistency is too thick, add the reserved water from the coconut cream 1 tablespoon at a time to thin.

Serve immediately in a cold glass, dusted with cocoa powder.

Store leftovers in an airtight container for up to 5 days in the refrigerator.

UTRITION: Cal: 126 | fat: 11.9g | protein: 0g | carbs: 3.1g | net carbs: 2.0g | fiber: 1.1g

Prep time: 20 minutes | Cook time: 2 hours | Serves 12

INGREDIENTS:

Unsalted butter, for greasing

6 tablespoons coconut flour

4 ounces (113 g) full-fat cream cheese, at room temperature

½ cup golden flaxseed meal, re-ground in a clean coffee grinder

2 large eggs

1 tablespoon granulated erythritol–monk fruit blend

1 teaspoon baking powder

⅛ teaspoon salt

6 tablespoons heavy whipping cream

¼ cup water

2 tablespoons unsalted butter, at room temperature, plus more for greasing

¾ cup heavy whipping cream

2 tablespoons water

2 large eggs

¼ cup granulated erythritol–monk fruit blend

½ teaspoon vanilla extract

⅛ teaspoon salt

2 tablespoons unsalted butter, at room temperature

6 tablespoons allulose

¼ cup heavy whipping cream

¼ teaspoon salt

½ tablespoon dark rum or ¼ teaspoon rum extract

DIRECTIONS:

Preheat the oven to 350ºF (180ºC). Grease the baking sheet with butter and set aside.

In a large bowl, using an electric mixer on high, mix the coconut flour, cream cheese, flaxseed meal, eggs, erythritol–monk fruit blend, baking powder, and salt until just combined, stopping and scraping the bowl once or twice, as needed. Slowly add the heavy cream and water to the batter and mix until thoroughly combined.

Pour the batter into the prepared baking sheet and bake for 30 to 35 minutes, or until lightly browned. Allow the bread to fully cool, 15 to 20 minutes, and cut into 1-inch squares. Put the cubed bread in another large mixing bowl. Leave the oven on.

Grease another baking sheet generously with butter and set aside.

In the medium saucepan, bring the heavy cream and water almost to a boil, then reduce the heat and add the 2 tablespoons of butter.

In the medium bowl, whisk the eggs, erythritol–monk fruit blend, vanilla, and salt. Temper the egg mixture by adding 3 tablespoons of the hot cream mixture to it and mixing well. Stir the remaining cream mixture into the egg mixture.

Pour the cream and egg mixture over the cubed bread in the large mixing bowl, toss to coat, and pour everything into the buttered baking sheet. Using a spoon, press down the bread to ensure the liquid covers it.

Bake for 40 to 45 minutes at 350°F (180°C) or until the egg mixture has set and the top is lightly browned. Cool for 5 minutes.

Store leftovers in an airtight container in the refrigerator for up to 3 days.

In the small saucepan, brown the butter over medium-low heat, stirring constantly. The butter will begin to foam and bubble, and after 2 to 4 minutes, you should begin to see browned bits on the bottom of the pan. At this point, remove the pan from the heat and continue to stir until the butter begins to lightly brown to a golden amber color.

Add the allulose, heavy cream, and salt to the browned butter and stir until well combined. Simmer over low heat for 15 minutes. Resist the urge to stir. At the 15-minute mark, turn off the stove and add the rum. Note that the sauce will foam up when you add the rum. Stir and turn the heat to low and allow the sauce to cook for another 10 minutes without stirring. This will thicken the sauce and cook down the alcohol.

To serve, cut the bread pudding into 12 slices and pour the rum sauce over each slice.

Store leftover sauce in an airtight container in the refrigerator for up to 3 days.

NUTRITION: Cal: 325 | fat: 32.0g | protein: 5.0g | carbs: 7.1g | net carbs: 2.9g | fiber: 4.2g

Prep time: 10 minutes | Cook time: 0 minutes |
Serves 6

INGREDIENTS:

8 ounces (227 g) strawberries, sliced

¼ cup granulated erythritol–monk fruit blend; less sweet: 2 tablespoons

½ ounce (14 g) full-fat cream cheese, at room temperature

1 cup heavy whipping cream, divided

⅛ teaspoon vanilla extract

⅛ teaspoon salt

DIRECTIONS:

Put the large metal bowl in the freezer to chill for at least 5 minutes.

In a blender or food processor, purée the strawberries and erythritol–monk fruit blend. Set aside.

In the chilled large bowl, using an electric mixer on medium high, beat the cream cheese and ¼ cup of heavy cream until well combined, stopping and scraping the bowl once or twice, as needed. Add the vanilla and salt and mix to combine. Add the remaining ¾ cup of heavy cream and beat on high for 1 to 3 minutes, until very stiff peaks form.

Gently fold the purée into the whipped cream. Refrigerate for at least 1 hour and up to overnight before serving.

Serve in short glasses or small mason jars.

Store leftovers in an airtight container for up to 5 days in the refrigerator.

NUTRITION: Cal: 160 | fat: 15.9g | protein: 0.9g | carbs: 4.0g | net carbs: 3.0g | fiber: 1.0g

CPSIA information can be obtained
at www.ICGtesting.com
Printed in the USA
LVHW051100010621
689026LV00008B/1119